強身不老法

24 Section Brocade Qigong

Strengthen Body Longevity Method

Translated by Franklin Fick

Shen Long Publishing
shenlongpub.com

Shen Long Publishing
shenlongpub.com

Originally Published 1935

Disclaimer
This book is intended for informational purposes only. The author (s), translator (s), and publisher of this book disclaim all responsibility for any liability, loss, injury, or risk, personal or otherwise, which is incurred as a consequence, directly or indirectly from reading and or following the instructions contained herein.

Please consult your physician before starting any exercise program.

Table of Contents

Translator's Introduction

This book illustrates a 24 Section Brocade Qigong that was lost in China, but preserved in Japan. To reintroduce the art back into China, the author examined and translated the Japanese text and this set of exercises was published in 1935.

One of the most popular Qigong sets is the 8 Section Brocade Qigong. There are many different versions of this exercise set. I have also seen 6 Section Brocade, 12 Section Brocade, and a version with 32 exercises (which was originally 64 exercises before it was simplified). These sets are usually either Seated Sets or Standing Sets. This 24 Section Brocade contains both seated and standing exercises.

I feel that there is some Japanese influence on how the exercises are presented. Most notably, the seated exercises use the kneeling position, called Seiza in Japan. Although the exercises might not be presented exactly how they would have been practiced in China long ago, I feel practitioners will still find this information useful and interesting in their research.

I also think this book will be interesting to practitioners of Japanese arts who wish to research body training methods and energy training methods. The author of this book claims that these exercises were used by the Japanese Samurai as their body strengthening and longevity method.

"According to the original authors words, after practicing this method for 100 days, it can make the

tendons, channels, bones, and muscles of the whole
body reach the condition of being solid and strong, the
activity of blood circulation increases, and it can make
the putrid that is stored inside the body exit completely
and all sorts of diseases will not be generated. After
practicing for 3 years, your strength will grow by 1000
times. The muscles are strong and solid like iron. No
matter where, even using knifes and swords to stab and
hack, one can not be hurt."

Introduction

This is a type of Wai Gong (external training). This is the
old method of 24 Section Brocade. It came from the
Shaolin External Family and later it was copied and passed
on to the outside and it was received by the Japanese
people. After they organized it and changed it slightly, then
it was given to the people. This is the Strengthen the Body
Longevity Method of the Samurai.

Actually this method came from our country. Most have
forgotten about our ancestors, almost to the point that it is
hidden. Never the less, today in our country the true
method of this old 24 Section Brocade has been long lost.
If you want to seek this true method, but you don't know
anyone who know it, there are one or two published
versions. Even though they are named 24 Section Brocade,
they came from other books, they are used to cheat people
to make easy profits, and they are not as organized as the
Japanese version of Strengthen the Body Longevity
Method.

Japanese people place the highest importance on Chinese
martial arts and they collect the ancient Chinese versions
especially. Which is why this version of 24 Section
Brocade has been passed on in Japan. I received the

8

original Strengthen the Body Longevity Method and studied its theories. It has places you must pay close attention. It is not as simple as average body exercises. I carefully translated the original text and I also drew its movements according to the pictures. When you read it it will be easy to understand completely.

According to the original authors words, after practicing this method for 100 days, it can make the tendons, channels, bones, and muscles of the whole body reach the condition of being solid and strong, the activity of blood circulation increases, and it can make the putrid that is stored inside the body exit completely and all sorts of diseases will not be generated. After practicing for 3 years, your strength will grow by 1000 times. The muscles are strong and solid like iron. No matter where, even using knifes and swords to stab and hack, one can not be hurt. The evidence is seen in many who practice this technique, the greatness of its effects. These are not empty words.

When I was translating and editing, I heard that the 24 Section Brocade has been passed on outside the country and we have not received its true version. That is why, I want to translate everything according to the original text and not mix in my own intention. Also, I do not want to consider myself clever and add and change to this book. (Doing that the result would be) to fool myself and others and to confuse the words and steal the name. As to the effects of this Strengthen the Body Longevity Method, if each section's movement is good or not, I would like to discuss and research with those who want to practice.

Ti Anshi

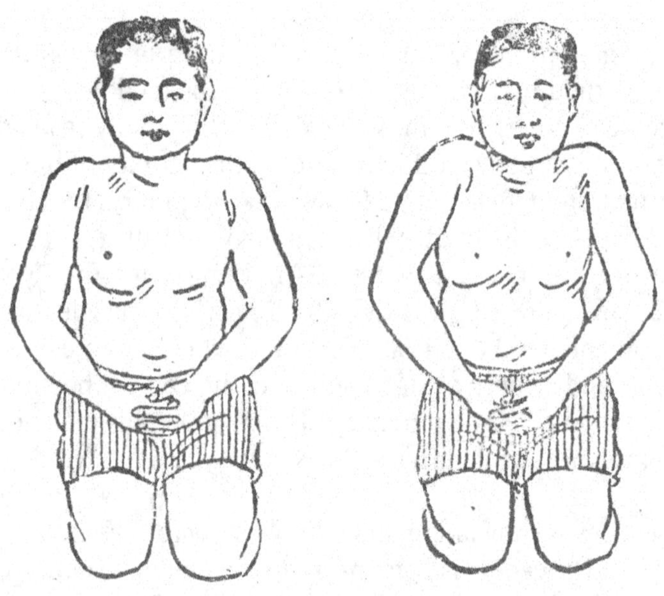

Picture 1

10

Section 1

Guiding Up and Down with Lower Abdominal Breathing about 24 times

Preparation

Face forward. Kneel in an upright posture. Connect the two knees and the big toes of the two feet. The fingers of the two hands are crossed and connected below the umbilicus, near the root of the thighs. The two elbows are close to the torso, so that the connected hands form an embracing posture.

Exercise

Close the mouth. Inhale through the nose. At the same time, the two shoulder rise upward. Exhale through the mouth and quietly return to the previous position. When the shoulders go up and down, it counts as 1 time. Repeat for about 20 times. The breathing must not have any sound. See picture 1.

Explanation

The speed of this first movement should be about the same as the breathing, which is about 1 second. It (the movement) must be quick and with force when guiding up and down.

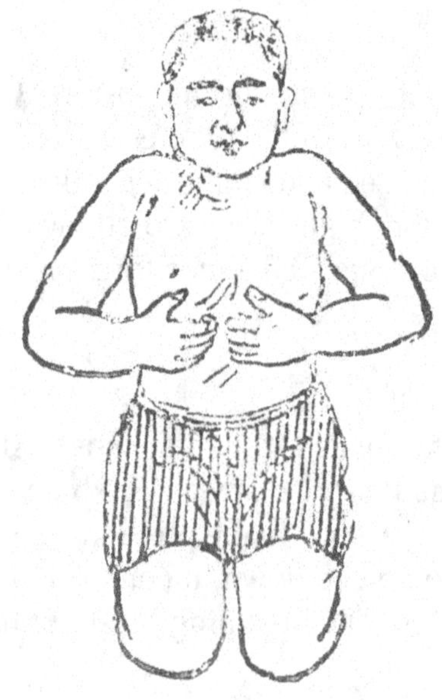

Picture 2

Section 2

Two Hands Embrace the Floating Ribs, Breath Deeply and Move the Shoulders Up and Down about 20 times

Preparation

Kneel the same as in the first exercise. The two palms embrace right below the V shaped bone (V shape of the ribs at the solar plexus). The tip of the fingers insert slightly into the soft part. The thumbs are positioned right below the nipples. Open the two upper arms. If the tendon is hard and you can not insert your fingers, then just point the fingers straight.

Exercise

The breathing is the same as the first exercise. At the same time (as the inhale), the two shoulders rise up together. Then immediately return to the previous position. This counts as 1. Repeat for about 20 times. The speed is the same as the first exercise. The breathing can not have any sound. See picture 2.

Explanation

This exercise moves the monk's hat tendon (trapezius). It has the function of guiding and extending the lungs and also increases the circumference of the chest.

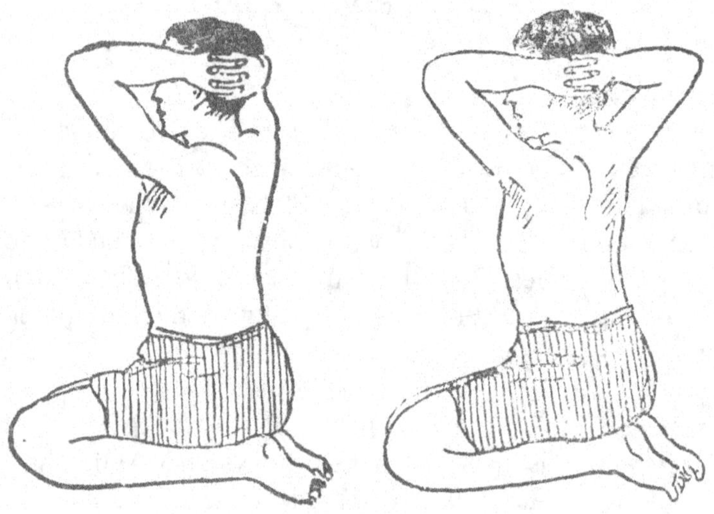

Picture 3

Section 3

Two Hands Connect Behind the Neck, Open and Close the Two Upper Arms about 20 times

Preparation

Kneel as in the previous two exercises. The ten fingers cross and embrace behind the neck. The tips of the two elbows face forward and are positioned below the two ears and where the wrists and the palms connect. The upper body is upright. Do not turn the body.

Exercise

The two elbows open to the left and right quickly and with force. The arms form one straight line and the two shoulder blades open until they touch each other. The elbows are level with the shoulders. Without pausing, return to the preparation posture. Repeat 30 times. See picture 3.

Explanation

This movement can make the left and right circumference of the chest increase evenly and also increase the top of the lungs. It also has the effect of increasing the elasticity and softness of all the muscles and tendons of the chest.

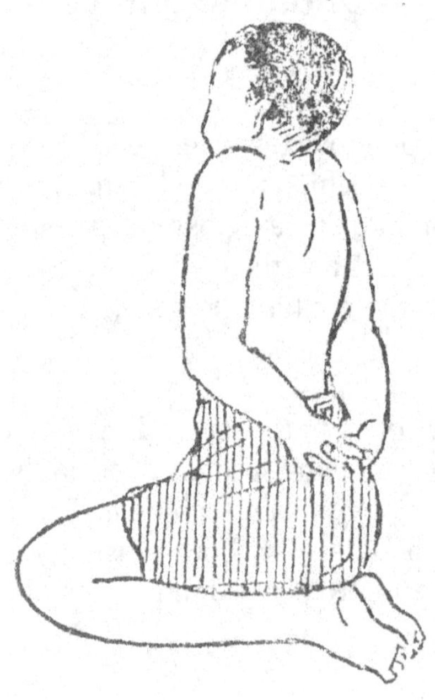

Picture 4

Section 4

Two Hands Connected in the Middle of the Back, Deep Breathing Move the Shoulders Up and Down about 20 times

Preparation
Kneel as previously. Move the two hands to the back. Firmly cross the fingers at the waist but do not use force. Allow the wrists to drop down.

Exercise
Inhale through the nose. At the same time let the wrists drop down and the shoulders go up. Then keep still. Then guide back downwards. The speed is the same as exercise 1 and 2. Repeat about 20 times. The breathing can not have any sound. See picture 4.

Explanation
Connecting the two hands in the back makes the posture upright and the movement can make the top of the lungs stretch vertically.

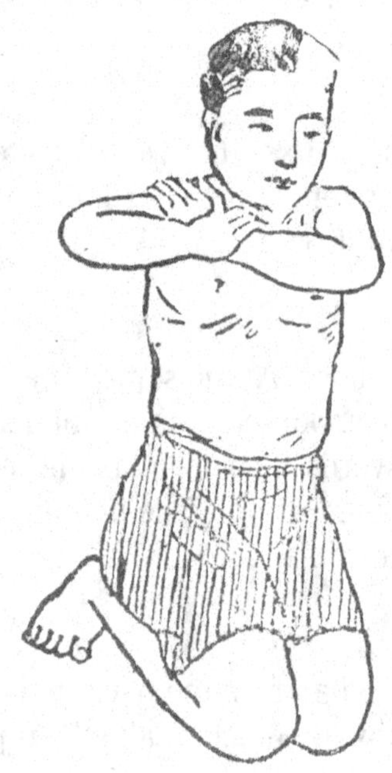

Picture 5

Section 5

Expanding the Circumference of the Chest, Move Left and Right about 10 times

Preparation
Kneel as previously. First bend the left wrist and place the hand on the right shoulder and touching the neck. The left arm is in front of the jaw and the wrist is level. The right palm tightly holds the middle of the left arm. The right wrist is at the height of the level line (of the left arm).

Movement
Use the right hand to pull the left arm to the right side with force, from the left upper arm to below the jaw. Then use opposing force to pull and guide the right wrist and arm. Strongly press to the left side, from the right upper arm to below the jaw. Then return to the preparation position. Continue left and right, each 10 times. See picture 5.

Explanation
The goal of this exercise is to completely open and shut the shoulder blades to the left and right and to make the chest area increase in size.

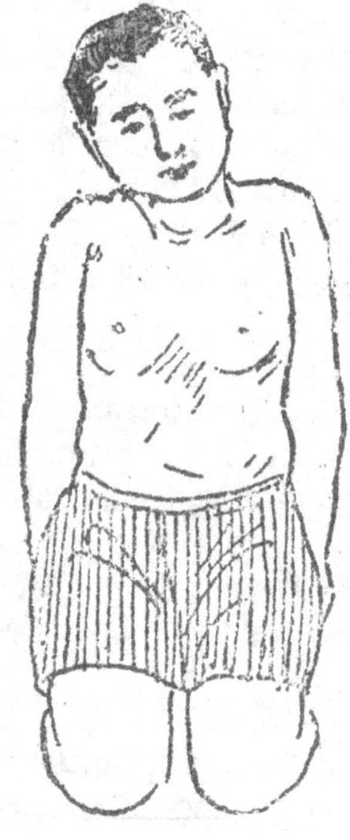

Picture 6

Section 6

Move the Head Left and Right, left and right combined about 12 times

Preparation

Kneel and face forward as previously. The two hands are dropped to the left and right. The head leans to the left.

Exercise

First move the head to the right shoulder and vibrate. When you guide the ear tightly next to the middle of the shoulder, you vibrate quickly with force. Then use its reflex to go to the middle of the left shoulder, the same as previously. Repeat about 12 times. See picture 6.

Explanation

This movement can extend and lengthen the neck tendons.

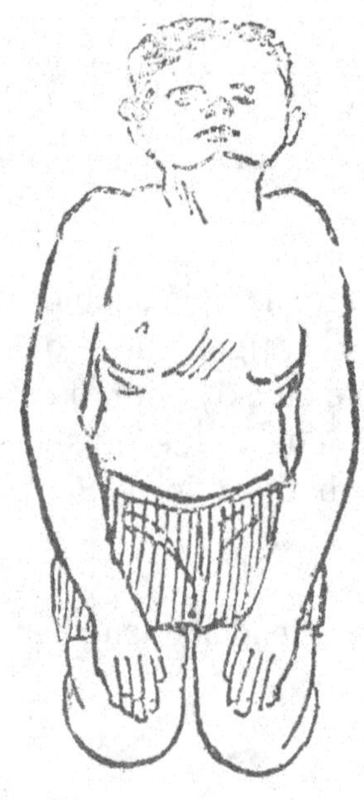

Picture 7

Section 7

Make the Head Vibrate Up and Down about 12 times

Preparation
Kneel as previously. The face is pointing upward. Put the two hands on top of the knees.

Exercise
First face downward and make the neck connect to the chest. Use its opposite force to immediately face upward and drop the head to the back. The back of the head should be connected to the back. Repeat this way 12 times. See picture 7.

Explanation
This exercise is for the whole neck. This will make the tendon of the head soft and thick. It can make the Monk's Hat Tendon (trapezius) and thyroid and the rest of the several tendons of the neck stretch and contract. It is very comfortable and at ease.

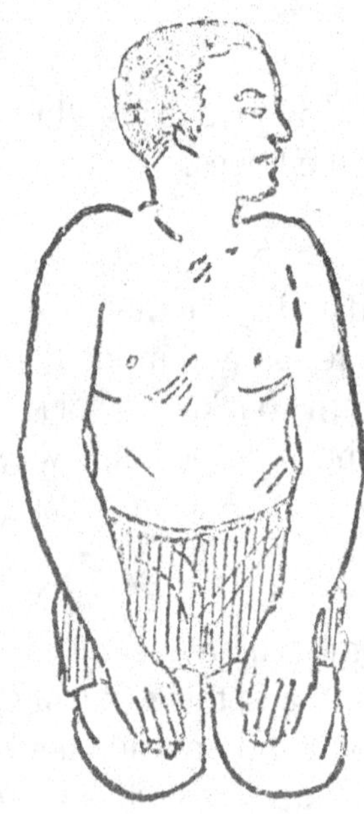

Picture 8

Section 8

Turn the Head Left and Right about 12 times

Preparation
The posture is the same as before, but the face is on top of the left shoulder

Exercise
First turn the head to the right. The jaw is on top of the right shoulder. Quickly vibrate with force. Then immediately turn the head to the left so the jaw is on top of the left shoulder. Repeat this way 12 times. See picture 9.

Explanation
This exercise is the same as the previous two exercises. It is to strengthen all the tendons of the neck and to make the joint of the neck move comfortably. It also has the effect of benefiting the ears.

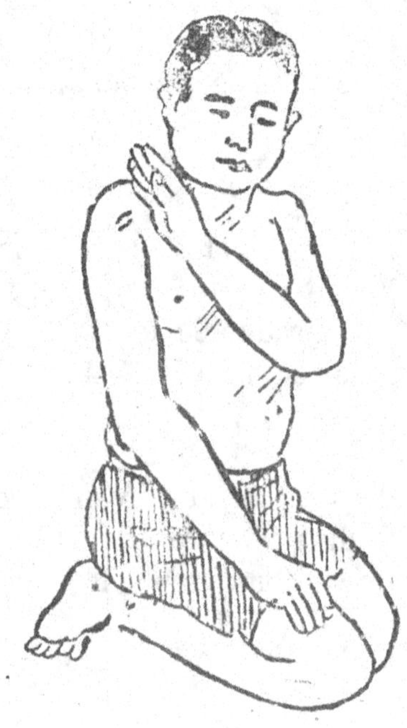

Picture 9

Section 9

Knock on the Neck about 6 times each

Preparation
Kneel as in the previous exercise. The head fully tilts to the left horizontally. The ear must touch the shoulder. Guide the left hand to the top of the shoulder. The thumb is bent and the four fingers spread open. The tip of the ring finger is bent and placed on the neck.

Exercise
Put the tip of the fingers at the neck. Tap the lymph nodes below the left ear. Tap 6 times. Then guide upward and tilt the neck in a diagonal. Tap below the jaw 6 times. Then make the face look up and with the tip of the fingers tap below the jaw 6 times.

After you finish tapping with the left hand, tilt the head fully to the right side and use the tip of the right hand to repeat the exercise on this side. See picture 9.

Explanation
This exercise can help the blood circulation to the brain and at the same time can prevent and cure diseases of the ear and rotten teeth. Also, tapping the upper part of the throat will strengthen the thyroid gland, teeth, and gums.

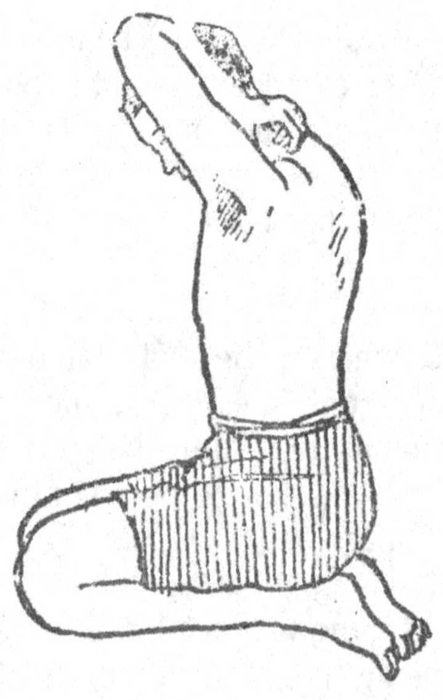

Picture 10

Section 10

Knock Behind the Head about 6 times

Preparation
Kneel as in the previous exercise. The head fully drops to the front. Place the tip of the little finger of the left hand behind the neck.

Exercise
Use the tip of the left finger, placed behind the neck, to tap 6 times at the sunken place behind the neck. Then raise the upper arm high to make it line up with the back of the neck. Then use the little finger of the right hand to tap 6 times in the same place. See picture 10.

Explanation
This exercise can prevent the spasm or paralysis of the facial nerves. It can also cure this type of disease.

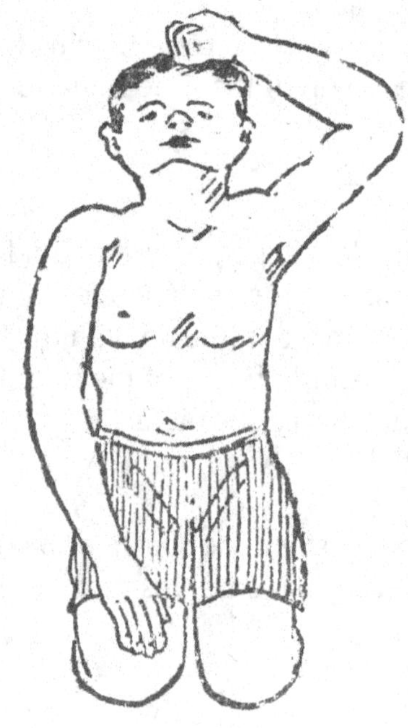

Picture 11

Section 11

Knocking the Face about 6 times

Preparation
Kneel and face upward. Drop the head fully to the back.
First make a fist with the left hand and place the fist on the
forehead.

Exercise
First use the left fist to tap the forehead 6 times. Then use
the right hand, following the same method, to tap 6 times.
See picture 11.

Explanation
Doing this exercise can prevent nasal puss, inflammation
of the nose, etc.

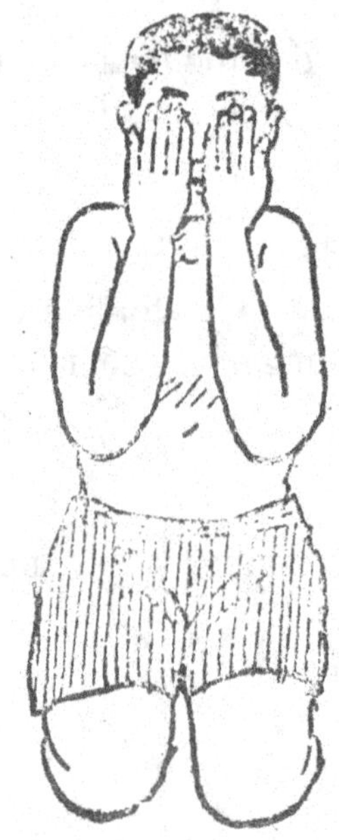

Picture 12

Section 12

Move the Eye about 2 times

Preparation
Kneel as before. Use the two hands with the ring finger and the middle finger touching each other. Each is placed at the space between the eyeball and the upper eye bone.

Exercise
With the fingers touching each other, use the fingers to press on the eyeball. Then move the fingers to between the eyeball and the lower eye bone and also press once. Then move the middle finger to the tip of the eye and the ring finger at the corner of the eye and also press once. Now, with the two palms supporting the checks and the two fingers tightly next to each other, press the middle of the eyeballs. Pressing 4 times this way counts as 1. Do this movement 6 times. See picture 12.

Explanation
This exercise can prevent nearsightedness and also has the ability to cure eyeball fatigue.

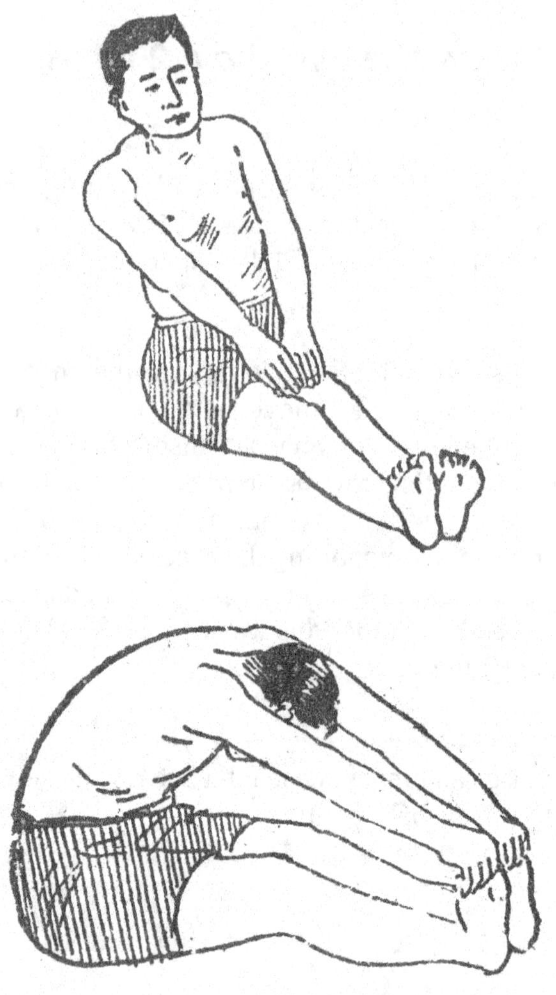

Picture 13

Section 13

Two Feet Straighten to the Front, Two Hands Stretch Out to the Front about 20 times

Preparation

Straighten the two legs out to the front. The tips of the feet face upward. The thumb of the two hands is placed on top of the knees. The upper body and the head move at the same time. Extend the wrists.

Exercise

First the two hands reach up over the upper body and then to the toes. Reach to the front quickly and with force. Utilize the opposing movement and immediately return to the previous posture. This counts as 1. Do this 20 times and stop. See picture 13

Explanation

This exercise can guide the tendons in the spine and prevent the bent waist and slouching posture of old age.

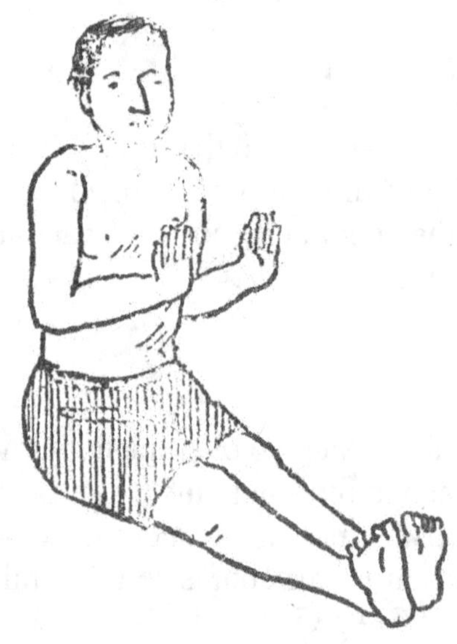

Picture 14

Section 14

The Whole Body Up and Down about 10 times

Preparation
Raise the two arms and straighten them to the front. The palms face each other and the distance between them is equal to the width of the shoulders. Do not form a V shape. The legs are tightly next to each other and the toes point upward.

Exercise
The elbows bend and return (to the body). The upper arm is next to the ribs. The forearm are level. The tips of the fingers face up and the palms face each other, as previously. From this posture, return to the previous position. This counts as 1 time. You must repeat this 10 times. See picture 14.

Explanation
This exercise can bring about the balance of the whole body and the regulation of the communication of the whole body. At the same time, it strengthens the abdominal tendons and increases the power of the shoulders and arms.

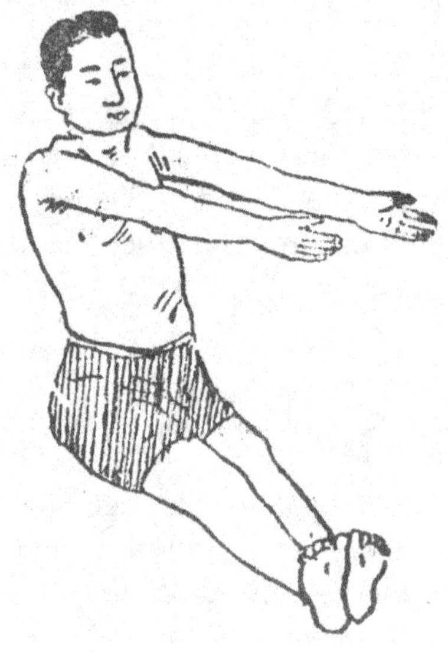

Picture 15

Section 15

Evenly Stretch and Straighten the Tendons on the Surface of the Abdomen and Correct the Bone Structure about 20 times

Preparation

The posture is the same as the previous exercise, Section 14, with the legs straightened and with the same position and direction of the hands.

Exercise

Raise the head completely. At the same time, the upper body goes backward with the most power. The two hands do not move. Stretch and guide the tendons of the chest and abdomen fully. This counts as 1. Repeat this 20 times. See picture 15.

Explanation

This exercise has the purpose of guiding and stretching the many tendons of the chest and abdomen.

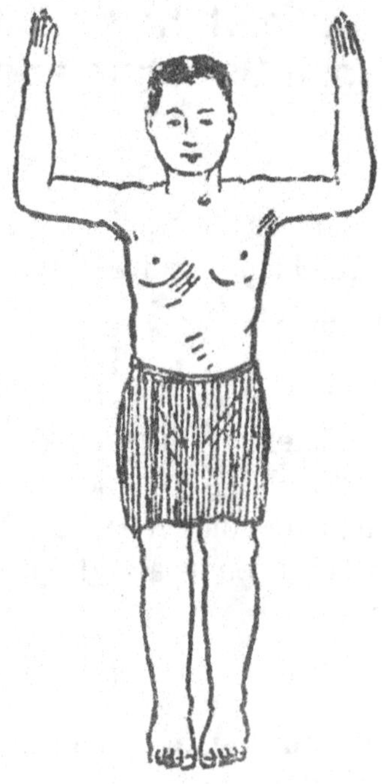

Picture 16

Section 16

Stand Straight, Move the Upper Arms Together to the Left and Right about 20 times

Preparation
Stand up straight and face forward. The feet open to a 60 degree angle. Drop the two hands to the outside of the hips.

Exercise
Raise the two hands to the front of the face. The bring them upward. The upper arms passes by the ears with the elbow straight. When they are at the back, they drop down. Do this 20 times. See picture 16.

Explanation
This exercise improves the activity of the Heart and promotes the circulation of the blood.

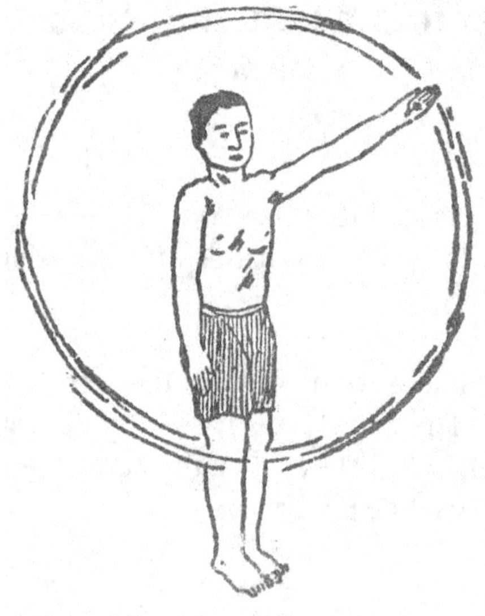

Picture 17

Section 17

Moving the Arms, Turning Up and Down, left and right each about 10 times

Preparation

Standing straight as in the previous exercise. Stretch the left wrist to the front, level with the shoulder. The ten fingers tightly close to form a fist.

Exercise

First the fist presses down and then turns to the back. Twist the shoulder and move to return to original position. This completes a big round circle. This counts as 1. The left hand moves 10 times. Then the right hand, using the same method, moves 10 times. See picture 17.

Explanation

This exercise makes the shoulder joint agile and also effects the tendons around the area.

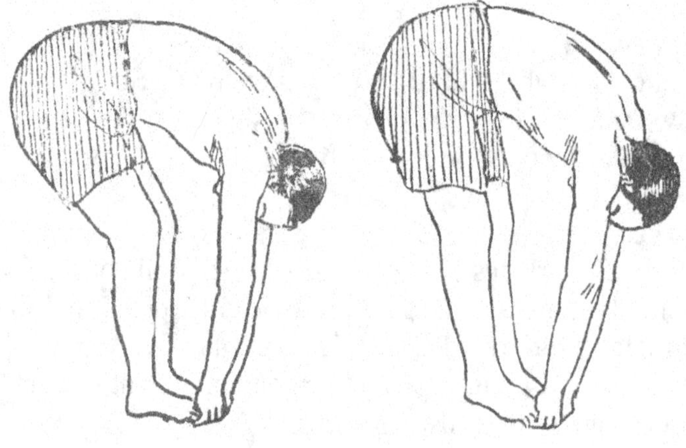

Picture 18

Section 18

Two Hands Grab the Toes, Move the Waist Up and Down about 10 times

Preparation
First bend the two knees to the front. Then the upper body leans down. Use the 4 fingers of the two hands to grab the tips of the toes of the two feet. Bend the knees to about 60 degrees. The toes step on the fingers. The fingers guide the feet up. Drop the neck. Do not bend the arms.

Exercise
Use the posture and raise the waist. The knees also stretch and straighten. Then return to the previous posture. This counts as 1. Repeat this 10 times. See picture 18.

Explanation
This exercise can open up the channels of the whole body and has the effect of clearing fatigue.

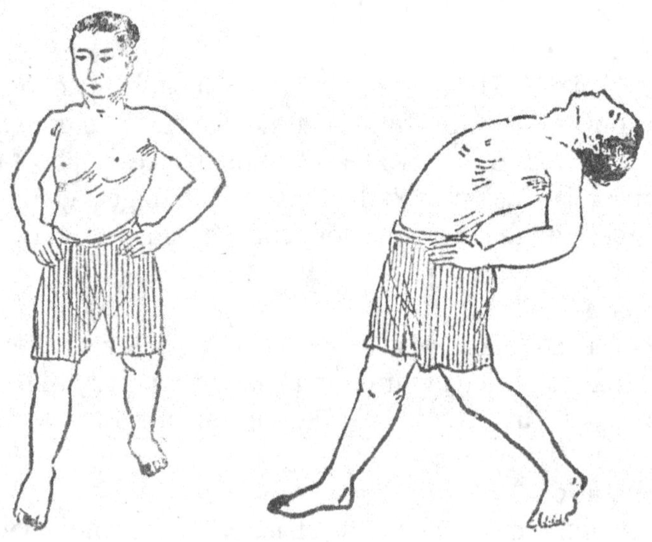

Picture 19

Section 19

Step Foot Forward One Step, Upper Body Bends Backwards, left and right each 6 times

Preparation

Stand up straight with the tips of the feet open. The left foot is placed at a 45 degree angle and the right foot points straight to the front. Step out about the distance of 1 ½ steps. The upper body and the left foot are facing in the same direction. The arms are bent at the elbows with the hands on the hips. The heel of the front and back feet must be on one straight line.

Exercise

First the upper body turns to the right. Then the upper body bends to the back. Then straighten the upper body and return to previous position. This counts as 1. Repeat this 6 times. Then change the position of the two feet and follow the method to repeat 6 times. See picture 19.

Explanation

This exercise can get rid of the congealed blood of the internal organs, increase the circumference of the chest, and exercise the stomach tendon, spine and marrow.

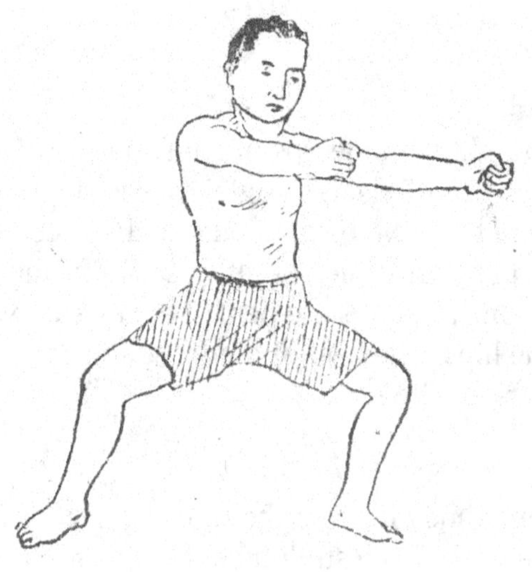

Picture 20

Section 20

Open the Legs and Bend at the Middle of the Waist about 20 times

Preparation

Stand up straight. The two legs point to the outside and open to about 80 degrees. The two hands are dropped down.

Exercise

First form the diagonal horse stance to the front. The hands form a tight fist. Raise the hands to the front with force. After a short while they drop down and return to the original position. This counts as 1. Repeat this 20 to 30 times. See picture 20.

Explanation

This exercise increases the ability of the stance.

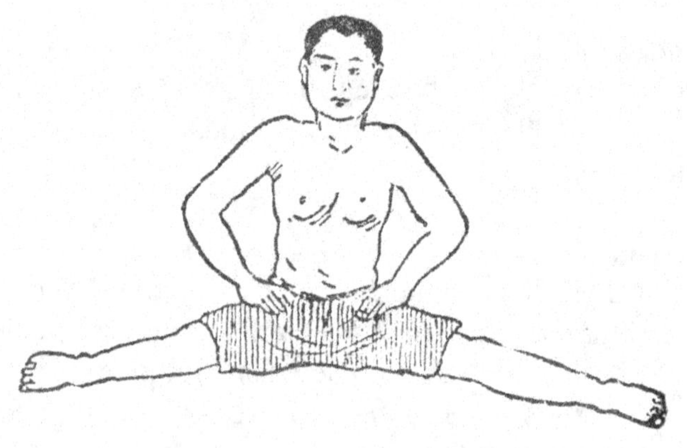

Picture 21

Section 21

Open the Legs to the Utmost Left and Right 2 times

Preparation

Stand straight. Bend the two arms and place them at the waist.

Exercise

Open the legs to the outside left and right. When you reach the utmost, the two legs form one straight line. It is best to make the thigh and the lower leg touch the floor. Then return to the previous position. Repeat this 2 times. See picture 21.

Explanation

This exercise is a type of riding the horse technique practice.

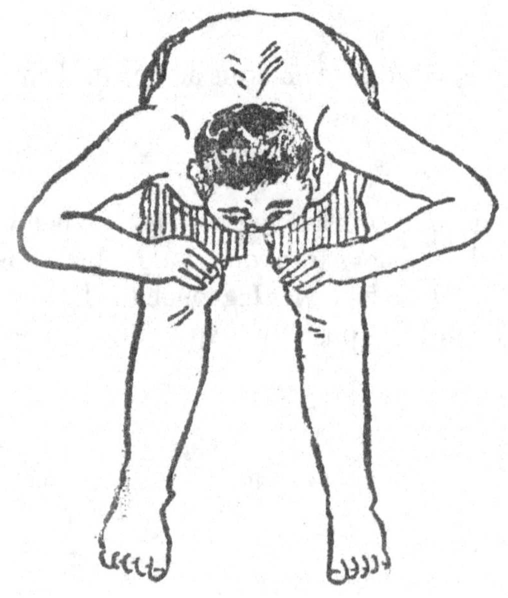

Picture 22

Section 22

Guide and Stretch the Spine about 20 times

Preparation
The legs open to the outside. The upper body sinks down. The palms press on the knees. The arms fully stretch to the outside. The shoulders are raised. The head tilts back. Slightly lean towards the back.

Exercise
Use the weight of the whole upper body to press down to the front. Make the waist as low as possible. Then immediately use the opposite force to return to the original posture. This counts as 1. Quickly repeat this 20 times. See picture 22.

Explanation
This exercise can correct a bent spine and also increases the circumference of the chest.

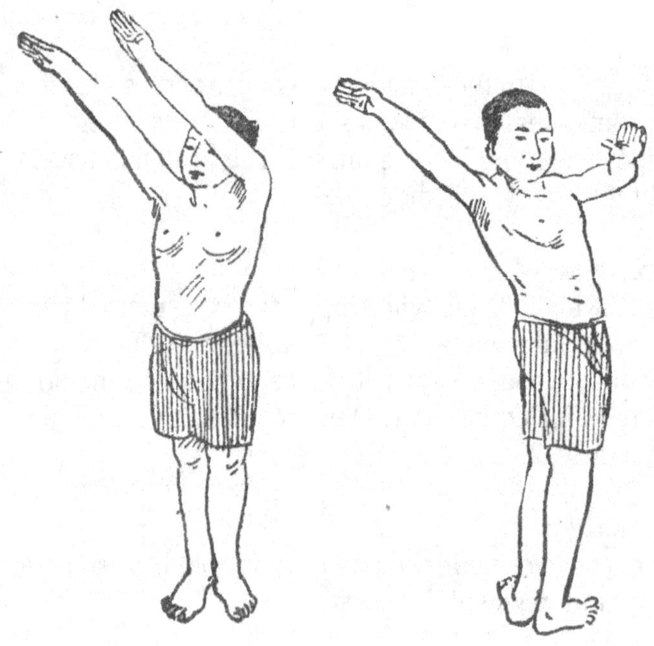

Picture 23

Section 23

Standing Straight Flap the Two Wrist to Make the Upper Body Turn Left and Right 20 times

Preparation

The body is upright and the heels of the two feet are about 3 cun (inches) apart. The left and right arms are raised upward. The upper body turns to the left. The backs of the hands face up and the palms face down.

Exercise

First turn the waist to the right. The right arm is level to the right and the left arm is level and bent to the front. The head turns to the right. The eyes look to the right. Do this 10 times, then change the position from left to right and repeat 10 times. See picture 23.

Explanation

This exercise can allow the body to change at will and also avoid danger.

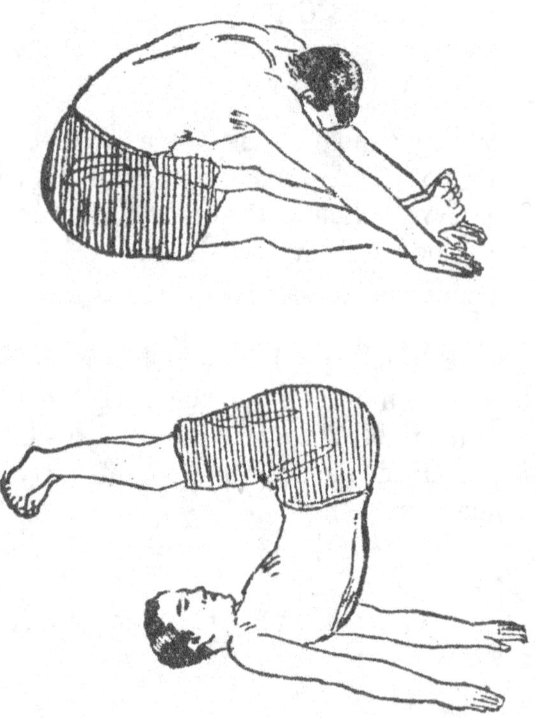

Picture 24

Section 24

Turn the Whole Body and Guide and Stretch the Spine to Increase Blood Circulation about 10 times

Preparation

Stretch and straighten the legs to the front. The upper body and head bend forward. The hands press on the floor next to the two feet. The knees are fully straightened.

Exercise

The two arms and upper body, with the most power, turn to the back, like you are laying down flat. The two legs, with the most force, raise toward the back and move over the head. At this time, only the head and the shoulders are touching the ground. After a short while return to the original position. Do this 10 times. See picture 24.

Explanation

This exercise helps the body to mature and develop and increases blood circulation.

About the Translator

Franklin Fick is a long time practitioner and teacher of Traditional Chinese Kung Fu, Qigong, Meditation, and Healing Arts. He also has a Masters Degree in Acupuncture and Traditional Chinese Medicine.

Sifu Fick has been offering Online Lessons since 2010. For more information please visit:

spiritdragoninstitute.com

About Shen Long Publishing

Franklin founded Shen Long publishing in 2005 with the goal to provide the best information and learning materials related to: Traditional Chinese Martial Arts, Qigong, Meditation, and Traditional Healing.

For a complete listing of our products please visit Shen Long Publishing's website at:

shenlongpub.com